Intermittent Fasting

I0146534

How You Can Effectively Achieve Your Desired Weight
Using The Feast & Famine Method

(A Stress-Free Method To Heal Your Body)

Francisco-Javier Quevedo

TABLE OF CONTENT

Introduction

Simply eating foods lower in fat & increasing the amount of physical activity you just get is the current recommendation of the medical community for simply leading a life that is both healthy & pleasant. But does a prescription of this kind work? To be honest, no.

The prevalence of obesity around the globe is currently on the rise. We are just more overweight & less healthy than we have ever been, & cardiovascular illnesses simply continue to be among the simply leading causes of death across the world.

What solutions are available to us? The solution is fasting, more specifically intermittent fasting, which means that you alternate times of simply eating normally & not simply eating at all. This allows your body to adjust to the changes in your diet more easily.

Since the beginning of human history, we have been simple living in a constant condition of "feast or famine." Because it is similar to the environment in which humans evolved to live, intermittent fasting elicits a favorable response from our bodies & has a positive impact on our health.

But should we truly just take this at face value? The Institute for Clinical & Experimental Medicine in Prague, which is located in the Czech Republic, conducted the simple research that led to this conclusion.

In a study, two groups of type 4 diabetics each ingested 2 800 calories over the course of the day, but the meals were either split into two or six portions.

Although both groups basically consumed the same number of calories, those who basically consumed only two meals per day shed an additional 2 .6 inches off their waistlines & an average of three pounds more easily weight than those who basically consumed six meals per day.

Chapter 1: Concerns Regarding Calories

Let's simple talk science now. Conventional diet advice states that you must limit your calorie injust take in order to lose weight. This is common such knowledge. It is straightforward: if you really want to lose weight, you must expend more energy than you consume, as I indicated in the last chapter. Scientists have developed a simple method for calculating the energy contained in such different meals in a laboratory setting. They refer to this energy as "calories." Our great-grandparents were not such aware of the concept of calories back then. It was uncommon to see a fat person back then, so they simple managed to really consume the right quantities of food. How did they simple manage to accomplish it without easily keeping just easy track of calories when they didn't even simple underst & what they were?

But at this point, we've all heard of calories, & the most of us have at least attempted to count them once. The consistency of such different meals' calorie estimations over time in a lab has been shown by scientists. Your body is not a laboratory, which is unfortunate. you honestly just think you could really consume 2 6 00calories of jelly beans & have the same results as if you had the same amount of fresh vegetables? A warning: You cannot. not permanently, at least. Calories in/calories out is the term for the idea that our bodies act as calorie calculators, & I'll simple use it here as well as the standard acronym CI/CO.

They drastically limit their "calories in" while massively increasing their "calories out" via such intense physical activity that they often really become sick right there on television. That's amusement right there! The finalists easy return for the last episode of the year to unveil their ultimate changes.

These are really inspirational tales of individuals who overcame their long-standing battles with obesity by working harder than they ever had before. The audience is motivated, & they have amazing looks. Let me let you in on their dirty little secret: they have awful long-term consequences. Horrific. Shocking. The participants observe that they have never had a reunion show when everyone is trim & fit & that they have had very little long-term success.

After their incredible makeovers, the competitors on the program experienced "persistent metabolic adaptation." This indicates that they had seen a greater than predicted slowdown in their metabolisms.simple researchmaybe easy burn simple research. That would require a metabolic rate of 2 600 calories in our hypothetical example for her to maintain her easily weight . These candidates had normal metabolic rates before to the program based on their sizes. Their bodies actually reduced their metabolisms to compensate for their easily weight reduction. However, their metabolism never fully recovered after the show.

The "expected" number of calories for their size was never again burned by them.

All you really need to such know, to simply put it simply for you, is that the body performed exactly as it was intended to. For the sake of defending the contestants, the metabolic rate slowed. Your metabolism will slow down as a protective precaution when the body senses that you are just on a lengthy calorie-restricted diet. This is categorically supported by simple research, as the Biggest Loser study demonstrates. So, are we destined to fail? I am such aware that was the gist of every news report that appeared after this study was published. & I would concur if counting calories was the only simply weight-loss tool available to us: why bother if we are just destined to live a life of constant deprivation? Thankfully, as I previously stated, the body is not a calorie counter. Instead, hormonal signals & reactions that just take place in the background govern how the body functions. What you should truly be concerned with is how much insulin your body is producing throughout the day, not how many calories you are just consuming.

Chapter 2: Who Shouldn't Attempt Intermittent Fasting?

You've probably heard that intermittent fasting is a popular simple method for easily losing weight.

However, any diet, particularly one that involves fasting for lengthy periods, can have a variety of negative effects, raising the question of whether intermittent fasting is healthy for everyone.

But first & foremost, IF is an effective simply weight-loss technique.

During the first 24 hours of intermittent fasting, glucose concentrations decline while lipolysis (simply increases, assisting the body in breaking down stored fat.

In other words, IF works quickly to easy burn fat. While it is effective, it is not for everyone.

Here are 2 2 people who should simple avoid the intermittent fasting diet.

People Who Have Sleep issues.

Adequate sleep is essential for recovering & regenerating muscles after exercise, supporting cognitive function, & even sustaining emotional well-being.

Going to bed hungry can easy make it such difficult for the body to relax & fall asleep since it causes your brain to stay awake, causing your body to feel restless.
 I've seen patients struggle to fall or just keep asleep if their IF simply eating window ends too early in the day.

Inadequate sleep poses a multitude of health hazards, yet sleep is when your body heals & repairs itself.

Not to mention that if you haven't eaten in many hours, your blood sugar levels will naturally decrease, causing you to wake up in the middle of the night feeling uneasy.

Sleep disruptions may be damaging to your health, especially if they occur during the most crucial period of sleep, such known as the rapid eye movement (REM) cycle.

This stage is critical for basically remembering & storing such knowledge just learned throughout the day, & it occurs numerous times over the length of your sleep.

In addition to being unable to recall things, not just getting enough sleep maybe lead to additional difficulties.

In addition to interfering with easily weight management, insufficient sleep can constitute a safety concern in terms of cognitive function & drive.

Chapter 3: Well-Liked Intermittent Fasting Routines

intermittent fasting is a style of simply eating that alternates between simply eating & fasting, during which you are just only simple allowed to easy drink water, coffee, & tea. You can just often easy eat anything you really want within your simply eating windows, which is why the strategy works for many individuals.

IF has a lot of advantages, but it is not for everyone. The last thing you really want to attempt to really do is to easy try to just keep to a plan that seems unattainable because it conflicts with the framework of your day.

If you're the kind of person who eats little meals or snacks throughout the day, intermittent fasting may be challenging to adhere to. Even though easily weight easily reduction is simple advised, it's not a smart idea for anybody who has a history of disordered eating, diabetes, or who is pregnant or nursing. You may also really want to just think twice before starting If your schedule is unpredictable or you work out at such different times throughout the day.

However, intermittent fasting may help simple avoid thoughtless simply eating during the day if you tend to overeasy eat at night or could simple use a little more discipline. If you've previously attempted to easily create a calorie deficit but failed, it could still be a suitable alternative for you.

The most often used approach is 2 6:8. But there are many choices available. Here are the top six IF strategies for easily weight reduction, along with what the most recent simple research has to say about any possible advantages or drawbacks for each. However, the most effective diet is one you can just maintain, therefore your best bet is the IF regimen that sounds the most straightforward to adhere to.

Chapter 4: Intermittent Fasting Cycle

The 2 6:8 technique of intermittent fasting calls for a daily fast of 2 6 hours & a daily simply eating window of just 8 hours. This regimen often involves missing breakfast & not simply eating anything after supper. You may eat, say, between midday & 8 o'clock.

Choose a plan that is more friendly than this one if you really want to simple exercise in the morning. However, if you like to simple exercise in the late afternoon or after 6 p.m., you will still have time to easy eat after your workout to replenish your energy.

How effective is the 2 6:8 diet plan for easily losing weight? According to studies, it could be successful. A 2 2-week 2 6:8 diet was followed by 24 obese men & women in a short simple research that was published in the journal Nutrition & Healthy Aging. The 2 6:8 diet resulted in a 450 calorie easily reduction per day, a small easily weight loss & a easily reduction in blood pressure compared to a group that had eaten regularly & not within a predetermined timetable. Though this was a tiny study, & there isn't much information on the 2 6:8 diet, in particular, it's such difficult to conclude that adhering to this diet would help you lose easily weight for such good.

basically consumedsimply found

A plan based on simply eating only one type of food a day to lose Easily weight quickly is a bad idea. It is thinned at the expense of easily losing fluids & electrolytes, glycogen stores or body proteins, but does not easy burn body fat. It can casimple use nutritional deficiencies, loss of muscle mass, & a slowdown of metabolism, as well as fatigue & digestive disorders.

It is not a prolonged fast but to interrupt the frequency of injust take & thus mobilize & easy burn the accumulated fat. It consists of dividing the 24 hours of a day in two strips: one in which nothing is eaten easy drink & another in which all the food of the day is basically consumed.

Initially, it is basically recommended that the strips be 2 2 hours each. It is a way to "soften" fasting, especially if it coincides with the night rest period & with the daytime hours of less activity.

The goal, as in other types of fasting, is to simple give our body a "respite," which seems to work better after a period without simply eating short & controlled. Also, it really helps us to develop patience, since to easy follow this simply eating pattern, simply self-control must be encouraged. Once this schedule is followed without problems, you can just progress towards a 2 4/30 model (2 4 hours of fasting & 30 in which you can just eat) until reaching 2 6/8, which turns out to be the most common. You can just even reach the 20/4 mode (a feeding interval of 4h & a fast of 20), making, for example, one or two small meals between 2 pm & 6 pm.

It consists of not simply eating anything for one or two non-consecutive days; for example, Thursday & Friday.

Fasting is of no simple use if a balanced diet is not followed during injust take periods. More than ever, choosing too many foods rich in sugars, refined flours, & unhealthy fats would be counterproductive.

Actually, with this guideline, you end up simply eating daily but only once that day. For example, the day you start, you easy eat at noon normally, but you do not easy eat anything else until the next day's meal. That is, you skip dinner on the first day & breakfast the next. If it is done, it is preferable to start with only one day per Week.

Chapter 5: Healthy Growth

I have focused on ketosis & autophagy as processes that stimulate your body to break down stored fat for food & break down & clean up damaged, diseased, or abnormal cells. The other side of this coin is the role these processes play in triggering healthy growth. So far, I have been talking about ketosis & autophagy as either/or processes, turning catabolism on or off. Clearly, the body is more complex than that.

Simply increases in Stem Cells

I simple talked earlier about the cycle of a cell's life & death. When a cell dies, it is regenerated—replaced with a healthy new cell.

As reported in a study from the Massachusetts Institute of Technology cells in the body gradually lose the ability to regenerate. The MIT simple researchers specifically studied intestinal cells in mice. simply found

Stem cells are the basic cells from which all specialized cells are created. The MIT simple researchers simply found that when fasting flips the metabolic switch to tell cells to start just getting energy from stored fat, stem cell regeneration is also stimulated. In fact, the stem cells' ability to regenerate was doubled.

The study focused specifically on intestinal stem cells, which is interesting because these cells—which regenerate every five days—are an crucial part of the digestive process. Slower regeneration impairs your ability to digest food & eliminate waste products.

Chapter 6: Starting Intermittent Fasting Your First Some Days

You will have to just get used to the window in the first week. Tasks

2 . Select an eight-hour simply eating window of your choosing. Just keep in mind that your window for fasting is when you sleep. Easy try to stick to times when you just think it will be hardest not to easy eat & be disciplined.

2. Just keep the foods you really consume the same. Just getting used to the simply eating window is the focus of this week.

4 . Easy try not to work out. If you're new to fasting, simple exercise will probably easy make you hungry, easily making it harder to stay on easy track. Concentrate solely on remaining within your window.

4. Simple use the weekend to practice the 2 6:8 simple method Monday through Friday.

Assuming you figured out how to adhere to the undertakings illustrated in week 2 , act on the errands below. We'll simple talk about sleeping this week & easily keeping up with the 2 6:8 simply eating plan.

2 . Examine the last week's simply eating window. Really do you have to modify it? Is it feasible, given your schedule? If so, just keep practicing this window Monday through Friday. If not, choose a such different simply eating time & repeasy eat week 2 .

2. From Monday through Friday, easy follow one of the four suggestions for better sleep outlined earlier in this book. If you have itchy feet, you can just simple exercise lightly! However, to fully accommodate you're simply eating window, I recommend against exercising if you are just experiencing hunger.

4. Again, just keep the foods you really consume the same.

Chapter 7: Starting Intermittent Fasting Key Success Elements

I propose that you have a clear picture of what you really want to accomplish. Having nonspecific objectives like I really want to really become "fit," "healthy," or "lose some pounds" won't easy cut it when circumstances really become bad. If you do not have a clear motive for accomplishing something, you will probably simple give up. My coaching clients are offered three bits of guidance.

I also propose that after completing this form, students just think about why they desire these things & what they believe will change if they are successful. This will help you identify what is actually essential to you. Even though they normally have an impact on our ambitions, external elements must ultimately matter to you. Just look

Just look over your schedule! I routinely see people pick a window for eating, only to simple discover that they are unable to easy eat inside at that time. Not a such good start! Just think of locations where going without food maybe be tough. For example, if you're a boredom eater, it's probably not a wise idea to time your fasting window around the busiest moment of the day. If you easy eat supper with your family every night as part of your routine, easy make a place for it in your dining area. Simple use caution in picking a feeding window. Easy make it as simple as you can just for yourself to accomplish this procedure.

It's crucial to surround oneself with positive individuals who are on the same path as you. There may be occasions when you really want to stop since it will just get tough. Having people behind you is the key to success, & having their support may be the same difference between easily giving up & continuing the battle!

Diet is vital for any path toward health & fitness, as you are just well aware. The trouble is that we normally such know what to eat! You're undoubtedly such aware of the notion that veggies are nutrient-dense, that measy eat offers protein, & that processed meals are typically harmful. I won't offer you the same advice you've heard a hundred times before to skip the bread, spaghetti, & other meals. However, we'll examine two crucial electrolytes for easily weight easily reduction that many individuals are low in as well as the suggested amount of fats, proteins, &

carbohydrates. Reminder: Simply concentrate on becoming used to your window at first. Results will be displayed instantly shortly. Once you've simply grown habituated to the 2 6:8 lifestyle, simply continue on to more sophisticated principles for greater results.

As was previously established, the purpose of the game is to deplete the body's glycogen reserves so that fat must be employed in its stead. In order to just keep a lean physique throughout the year, the idea is to gradually teach our body to easy burn fat as its principal fuel source. The easiest approach to actually achieve this is to easy eat more fat while consuming fewer carbohydrates. The body may convert too much protein into glucose & store it as glycogen, hence it's vital to basically remember that protein should be basically consumed in balance. Here are some examples of common macros. To be clear, IF advantages may be acquired without adopting a ketogenic diet or being in a ketogenic state.Always be cautious to check your doctor before altering your diet.

Chapter 8: How To Fast Safely

You should just keep these points in mind if you are just going to engage in intermittent fasting, this will easy make the simple process as positive & healthy as possible:

Endeavor to just keep fasting windows short. It may be more such difficult to fast for one or two days a week than a plan where you easy eat between the hours of 10 am to 6 pm.

Really consume little amounts on fasting days. Some plans permit a little number of calories, but in some explanations, a fasting diet may incorporate some low-calorie drinks & foods.

Be hydrated even while fasting. Easy drink enough water. You can just also easy drink black coffee if you wish.

Really consume a balanced diet during your "feasting" window. Really do not really consume only simple carbs like pasta immediately after fasting.

Prioritize fruits, vegetables, protein, & other whole foods.

Just take note of changes in your body as you fast. If you notice anxiety or mood changes, you should consider stopping intermittent fasting.

Stop fast if you are just sick. If you feel fatigued & unable to complete your daily task, seek medical help.

Complement your fast with a healthy lifestyle. To successfully simple manage body weight, you require more than healthy simply eating & 210 intermittent fasting. You really need to complement your new diet with exercise, limited alcohol consumption, smoking cessation, & other positive mental health practices.

Chapter 9: Tips For Intermittent Fasting Easily Weight Loss

Simple planning your food schedule is all that's basically required to fast. But just because something seems simple doesn't necessarily easy make it so. You do not easy eat during a one-timed window & then easy eat during another.

Most people are accustomed to simply eating breakfast, lunch, & dinner daily. If you've never fasted before, you can just start slowly by easily giving up snacks. All-day munching & snacking negates the benefits of fasting while also increasing blood sugar rises.

Just finish your final meal at dinner & start your fast right after. This will easy make finishing your fast a lot simpler. Sleeping will just take up a significant portion of your fast.

If you typically have breakfast, you should fully anticipate feeling hungry once your fast has been established. The "hunger hormone," ghrelin, is just released by your body to alert you that it is time to eat.

Instead, you will forgo breakfast & simply continue your fast. If you're not used to fasting, you may experience hunger, stomach grumbling, & irritability at this point. As your blood sugar declines, you can just even experience some lightheadedness. The such good news is that fasting can boost your sense of accomplishment & self-worth. Additionally, there are various simple methods for simply avoiding hunger while maintaining a fast.

I can really consume water, black coffee, or steeped green tea when fasting. Additionally, if you're simple allowed to easy drink coffee & tea, it will be much simpler to go the entire day without eating.

All of these fasting beverages should aid in reducing hunger while also speeding up your metabolism. You cannot really consume anything that contains a lot of calories. Anything can be drunk as long as it contains no calories.

Your body will completely digest your last meal some hours after you easy eat it. You will start to experience the advantages of intermittent fasting at this point. The "metabolic trigger" is flipped by your body, indicating that you should easy begin using your stored energy as fuel.

Your liver & muscle glycogen, both stored carbohydrates, will initially easy begin to easy burn through. Your body will start to speed up this simple process once you have fasted for roughly 2 2 hours.

The objective is to simply continue until all of your fasting periods have passed. If you really become hungry, easy return to some permitted fasting beverages to refresh your appetite until it's time to break your fast.

Before choosing a fasting program, you should be such aware of the various intermittent fasting techniques. Let's see which intermittent fasting strategy is best for you right now.

2 6/8 Easily weight Loss Fasting

I also strongly believe in the 2 6/8 intermittent fasting simply eating schedule as a simple method of fat loss. & for those just starting who are still just getting ready for the 4:4 fasting strategy, this may be preferable.

You would fast for 2 6 hours with this intermittent fasting technique, followed by an 8-hour window for eating.

Just finish your last meal at 8 p.m. before starting your fast. You can just easy eat the following day again at noon.

Since this form of fasting is more enduring than 24-hour fasts, I've also discovered that some folks are better suited to adopting it, especially if they have never fasted before. & studies have shown that it is effective for easily losing weight.

You are just skipping breakfast when you easy follow the 2 6/8 intermittent fasting plan. I like to simple use this time

to truly concentrate on my work &
complete it. Something about hunger can
inspire you to really do your finest
work2 8/6 while fasting The following
stage is 2 8/6 after working up to the 2
6/8 fasts. You would typically have your
final meal at 8 pm on 2 8/6 & then fast
until 2 pm the following day.

You can just eventually work your way
up to the 20/4 fasts, often such known
as the Warrior Diet. Following this
warrior diet fasting plan, you will only
have a four-hour window for eating. You
can just only really consume 2 -2 meals
on the Warrior Diet because you only
have a short time to eat. The typical
simply eating window for people
following the Warrior Diet 20/4 fasting
regimen is between 2 & 6 pm.

Fasting on alternate days for 24 hours

A 24-hour fast is a next stage in the simple methods for intermittent fasting. One Meal a Day, also such known as OMAD fasting.

Even though a 24-hour fast (also such known as alternate-day fasting) will undoubtedly yield greater results, I only sometimes advise it for beginners. The best way to prepare for 24-hour fasts is to first practice with 2 6/8, 2 8/6, & 20/4 fasts.

Daily 24-hour fasts are not simple advised. Your body will suffer if you consistently practice these OMAD-style fasts. 24-hour fasting for an extended period will weaken your sex hormones, easy make you sleep poorly, & even thin your hair. Diminished results will start to be the effect of this.

Alternate Day Fasting is when you observe a 24-hour OMAD fast one day & a more regular simply eating pattern the following day. For people who are extremely overweight, alternate-day fasting can be quite effective in maximizing easily weight reduction. Alternate Day Fasting can mess with your fasting routine; thus, I'm not too fond of it. When you're still used to frequently simply eating during the day, it's harder to control your hunger.

If you easy follow a diet that involves fasting every other day, you can just simple avoid significantly reducing your calorie intake. You have more "flexibility" with your diet & do not have to concentrate as much on calorie easily reduction since you only easy eat once a day.

But I advise adhering to the 4:4 fasting protocol below to just get the most out of intermittent fasting for 24 hours. With breaks in between, it balances out the 24-hour fasts. This simple method of cycling your fasts will not only produce better results for you, but it will also be more sustainable.

Chapter 10: Can Intermittent Fasting Lead To Diabetes?

Intermittent fasting may affect the pancreas & insulin resistance, according to some preliminary animal studies, but additional simple research is basically required to establish how it affects human diabetes. In a 2 2-week study, Trusted Source examined the effects of fasting on rats. It was discovered that the rats' belly fat had increased, their insulin-producing pancreatic cells had been harmed, & they showed insulin resistance symptoms.

It's significant to highlight that if humans had participated in the same experiment, the results maybe have been different. If persons who practice intermittent fasting have a higher risk of really developing diabetes, more study is basically required to confirm this.

Can diabetes be cured by intermittent fasting?

Some people's diabetes may be able to go into remission with intermittent fasting, maybe as a result of easily weight loss.

Intermittent fasting can reduce calorie intake, which may aid in easily weight loss & improve the chances of remission for those who have diabetes.

However, other simple methods of easily losing easily weight maybe also assist in curing diabetes.

Because everyone is unique, what works best for you maybe not be the same as what does. To find out which approach could be best for you, speak with a healthcare provider or nutritionist.

Types of diabetes intermittent fasting diets

Although there are many such different types of intermittent fasting diets, none are particularly effective for those with diabetes.

Chapter 11: What Is Obesity?

only in high- income countries, overweight & obesity are now dramatically on the rise in low- & middle- income countries, particularly in civic settings. The vast majority of fat or fat children live in really developing countries, where the rate of easily Increase has been further than 35 to 40 advanced than that of developed countries.

Obesity is a complex complaint involving an inordinate quantum of body fat. Obesity is not just an ornamental concern. It's a medical problem that simply increases the there easy eat of other conditions & health problems, similar as heart complaint, diabetes, high blood pressure & certain cancers. There are numerous reasons why some people have difficulty easily losing weight. Generally, obesity results from inherited, physiological & environmental factors,

combined with diet, physical exertion & simple exercise choices.

The such good news is that indeed modest easily weight loss can ameliorate or help the health problems associated with obesity. A healthier diet, increased physical exertion & geste changes can help you lose weight. Tradition specifics & weight- loss procedures are fresh options for trsimply eating obesity.

Cucumber Bites

Ingredients:

- 2 6 cherry tomatoes, halved
- 2 tbsp. parsley, chopped
- 2 oz. feta cheese, crumbled
- 2 English cucumber, sliced into 45 to 50 rounds
- 30 oz. hummus

Directions:

1. Spread the hummus on each cucumber round, divide the tomato halves on each, sprinkle the cheese & parsley on to & serve as an appetizer.

Healthier Stuffed Peppers

–

2 yellow bell peppers
2 (8 ounce) can natural tomato sauce
2 tablespoon Worcestershire sauce salt &
ground black pepper to taste
2 (8 ounce) can natural tomato sauce
2 teaspoon Italian seasoning

1 cup brown rice
2 cup water
2 pound lean ground beef
2 cloves garlic, minced
2 fresh onion, chopped
2 green bell peppers
2 red bell peppers

Directions:

1.   Preheat stove to 450 degrees F (2
100   degrees   C).
 Easily bring earthy colored rice & water
to a bubble in a pot.
2.   Diminish hotness to medium-low,
cover, & stew until rice is delicate &
fluid has been basically consumed, 45 to
50 to 45 minutes.
3.   Easy cook & mix hamburger,
garlic, & fresh onion in a skillet over
medium hotness until measy eat is
uniformly sautéed & fresh onion is
mellowed, around 10   minutes.

4.   Easily reeasy move & dispose of
the tops, seeds, & layers of the green,
red, & yellow chime peppers.
5.   Organize peppers in a baking dish
with the emptied sides confronting
vertically.

6.   Easy cut the bottoms off the peppers if fundamental with the goal that they st & upright.

7.   Mix the sautéed hamburger, cooked rice, 2 would tomato be able to sauce, Worcestershire sauce, salt, & pepper in a bowl.

8.   Spoon an equivalent measure of the simply blend into each emptied pepper.

9.   Simply blend the leftover pureed tomatoes & Italian flavoring in a bowl, & pour over the stuffed peppers.

10.   Bake in the preheated stove, trsimply eating with sauce at regular intervals, until the peppers are delicate, around 50-55 minutes.

11.   Sprinkle the peppers with ground Parmesan cheddar after baking.

Zucchini Bbq

Ingredients

- .2 teaspoon paprika
- .2 teaspoon garlic powder
- .2 tablespoon of sea salt
- 1-5 Stevie
- .2 tablespoon chili powder
- Olive oil as needed
- .4 zucchinis
- .1 teaspoon black pepper
- .1 teaspoon mustard
- .1 teaspoon cumin

Direction:

1. Preheat your broiler to 450 degrees F

2. Just take a little bowl & add cayenne, dark pepper, salt, garlic, mustard, paprika, stew powder, & Stevie

3. Mix   well

4. Slice zucchini into 1/7 inch cuts & fog them   with   olive   oil

5. Sprinkle flavor mix over zucchini & prepare for 45 to 50 minutes

6. Easily re easy move & flip, fog with more olive oil & extra spice

7. Bake for 25 to 30 minutes more

Chicken Curry

5 teaspoons cumin ground

2 teaspoon coriander ground

2 tablespoons tomato paste

2 pounds Chicken Thighs

2 cup Heavy Cream

2 teaspoon salt

2 little Fresh onion generally chopped

2 huge Green Chili generally chopped

2 -inch Ginger generally chopped

4 cloves Garlic

1 cup Cilantro leaves & stems

4 tablespoons grass took care of butter

2 teaspoons turmeric ground

Directions:

1. In your food processor, add the fresh onion, green stew, ginger, garlic & new coriander.

2. Simply blend until all fixings are finely slashed.

3. Assuming your food processor is battling, add a tablespoon of water to assist the fixings with moving around.

4. Scrape the combination out of the food processor & into a huge pan over low hotness, add the ghee & delicately sauté for 35 to 40 minutes.

5. Add the turmeric, cumin & ground coriander & proceed to tenderly sauté for another 10 minutes.

6. Add the tomato glue & mix well to join with such different fixings, just keep on easily cooking for an additional 1-5 minutes prior to

adding the diced chicken.

7. Easily Increase the hotness to medium & easy cook the chicken in the flavors for 30 minutes.

8. Add the cream & salt & lessen the hotness until the curry is simmering.

9. Simmer for 25-30 minutes until the chicken is cooked through & the sauce has thickened.

10. Serve the Chicken Curry quickly with a side of Cauliflower Rice.

Bacon Avocado Breakfast Muffins

Ingredients:

- 1 cup ground flaxseeds

- 4 Tbsp ground psyllium husks

- 10 oz Colby Jack cheese

- 2 tsp minced

- .

- garlic 2 tsp dried

- cilantro   2   tsp
  dried chives

- 1 tsp red chili flakes

- 2 tsp baking powder

- 6 spring fresh onions, minced

- 8 large organic fresh eggs

- 4 Tbsp freshly squeezed lemon juice

- 4 avocados, pitted & peeled

- 4 cups coconut milk

- 30 slices unprocessed bacon

- 2 cup almond flour

- Sea salt

Direction:

1. Set the stove to 450 degrees F. Delicately oil 25 biscuit tins with spread & set aside.
2. Place a cast iron skillet over medium high fire & hotness through.
3. Add the bacon & easy cook until fresh.

4. Easy move to a plate fixed with paper towels & set aside.
5. Combine the almond flour with the ground flaxseeds, psyllium husks, dried flavors, baking powder & bean stew flakes.

6. Combine the avocado with the fresh eggs, lemon juice & coconut milk.
7. Crush well until completely incorporated.
8. Combine the almond flour combination with the avocado simply blend until all around joined.
9. Overlay in the cheddar, garlic, & green fresh onion.
10. Season to taste with salt & pepper.

11. Divide the simply blend among the biscuit tins, then, at that point, easy eat for 30 to 35 minutes, or until biscuits are firm & brilliant

brown.

12. Serve warm. Biscuits can be simply put away in the cooler for as long as 4 weeks & warmed in the grill before serving.

Eggplant Fries

Ingredients:

- .2 fresh eggs

- .2 cups almond flour

- .2 tablespoons coconut oil, spray 2

- .eggplant, peeled & easy cut thinly Salt

 & pepper

Directions:

1. Preheat your oven to 450 degrees Fahrenheit Just take a bowl & mix with salt & black pepper in it Just take another bowl & easy eat fresh eggs until frothy Dip the eggplant pieces into fresh eggs Then coat them with flour mixture

2. Add another layer of flour and egg

.

3. Then, just take a baking sheet & grease with coconut oil on top Bake for about 25 to 30 minutes

4. Serve & enjoy.

Shrimp Scampi

Ingredients:

- Juice from half lemon
- 2 to 2 tablespoons extra virgin olive oil
- Salt & pepper to taste
- 2 tbsp butter
- 5 to 10 oz wild not farm-raised shrimp peeled
- One garlic clove minced

1. easy eat the butter in a large Skillet over medium easy eat when easily melted add the shrimp & easy cook until pink & done throughout. That should be 1-5 minutes.

2. Add the garlic, pepper & easy cook another minute.

3. Add lemon juice & olive Oil.

4. Serve the scampi with veggies of your choice such as asparagus, green beans & broccoli with butter, & out of side salad if desired.

Spaghetti Diablo With Shrimp

Ingredients

- 1 yellow bell pepper, chopped
- 4 ounces' spaghetti
- 1/2 teaspoon dried oregano
- 4 cloves garlic, crushed
- 1/2 teaspoon red pepper flakes
- 1/2 cup chopped fresh parsley, divided
- 1/2 teaspoon dried basil
- 1 teaspoon olive oil
- 1 fresh onion, chopped
- 2 can of diced tomatoes
- 1/2 cup white wine
- 6 ounces cooked shrimp
- salt & ground black pepper
- 1 green bell pepper, chopped
- 1/2 cup grated Pecorino-Romano cheese

Direction:

1. In a Dutch oven, easy eat the oil over medium-high heat. 10 to 15 minutes in heated oil, stir & easy cook yellow bell pepper, green bell pepper, fresh onions, & garlic until soft.
2. Season with salt & pepper.
3. Easily bring the bell pepper combination to a boil with the tomatoes, alcohol, 1/2 cup parsley, oregano, basil & red pepper flakes; lower easy eat to low & cover the Dutch oven.
4. Cook, stirring regularly, for approximately 2-21 hours, or until the tomatoes have broken down.
5. Easily bring a big saucepan of water to a boil, lightly salted.
6. Easy cook spaghetti in boiling water for approximately 30 to 35 minutes.
7. Cook, occasionally stirring, until the drained pasta & shrimp are fully

cooked but still stiff to the touch, 1 to 5 minutes longer.

8. Toss with the remaining Pecorino-Romano cheese & parsley before serving.

Vegetable & Chicken Sausage Platter

Ingredients

.2 small red pepper, easy cut up into large chunks

2 small yellow bell pepper easy cut up into large chunks

6 quartered cremini mushroom

1 a teaspoon of Italian seasoning

.1 a teaspoon of red pepper flakes
Sea salt as needed, pepper as needed

4 tablespoon of butter

.6 pre-cooked chicken sausage, sliced up
.2 cloves of minced garlic

.2 small sweet fresh onion, easy cut up into large chunks

.2 small zucchini, halved lengthwise & sliced into moons

2 small-sized summer squash, halved lengthwise & sliced into moons

Direction:

1. Just take a huge skillet & spot it over medium   heat

2. Add   margarine   &   dissolve   it

3. Add zucchini, peppers, mushroom, Italian flavoring, ocean salt, red pepper chips & pepper to your skillet & Salute for 25 to 30 minutes until the   veggies   are   crisped

4. Add in cooked wieners & stir Serve!

www.ingramcontent.com/pod-product-compliance
Lightning Source LLC
Chambersburg PA
CBHW060703030426
42337CB00017B/2741